The 5 Biological Laws

The Skin and Skin Allergies

Dr. Hamer's New Medicine

The 5 Biological Laws: The Skin and Skin Allergies

Dr. Hamer's New Medicine

ISBN: 9781500730581

For information and orders of the following book, you can contact the Author by following addresses:

www.5biologicallaws.com

to Matilde

Warnings

The author declines any responsibility for the information, and the use of the arguments dealt in this text. Nothing exposed here has to be meant to replace the academic and official medicine.

Today Official Medicine has not verified and recognized Dr. Hamer's discoveries.

We remember the reader this text does not want to replace some diagnosis and medical therapy, but the same has to apply to competent therapists in order to compare the benefits and the risks of the currently offered therapies.

Andrea Taddei

The 5 Biological Laws

Bones, Muscles and Articulations

Dr. Hamer's New Medicine

Index

Presentation

The 5 Biological Laws discovered by Dr. Hamer, they represent a new key of reading and understanding of all the defined processes called pathological.

This book, in particular, deals in a very in depth way the conflicts regarding the inherent conflicts of "separation" and "feeling attached".

Furthermore, they are explained from the point of view of the 5 Biological Laws, most common and diffuse pathologies regarding the skin system like: Acne Vulgaris, Angiomas, Alopecia , Alopecia Areata, Androgenic Alopecia, Callosity, Cellulite, Dermatitis, Eczema, Urticaria, Dyshidrosis, Genital Herpes Labial Herpes, Psoriasis, Nevi, Moles, Pediculosis, Skin Fungi, Sweating, Urticaria, Vitiligo, Warts, Zoster Herpes.

The New Germanic® Medicine, discovered by Dr. Ryke Geerd Hamer and systematized in the 5 Biological Laws, represents a change in the understanding of what is commonly called Disease.

Through his studies, Dr. R. G. Hamer has ascertained that the pathological processes are not "Biological errors of the nature" but Sensible Programs of the Nature consequent on very precise events.

1. The 5 Biological Laws

1st Biological Law of Nature

1st Criterion: every Significant Biological Special Programs of Nature (SBS) originates from DHS (Dirk Hamer Syndrome), with an unexpected conflict shock, acute and dramatic, lived intensely and with a feeling of isolation. Starting from DHS, every SBS manifests itself simultaneously on three levels: psyche, brain, organ.

2nd Criterion: DHS determines the location of the SBS both at brain level, the so-called Hamer Focus, and at organ level where it causes an organic alteration.

3rd Criterion: the course of the SBS runs synchronously on all three levels (psyche, brain and organ), from DHS to the resolution of the conflict (CL), including epi-crisis (CE) at the top of the Post-Conflict phase (PCL) until normal level is restored (normotonia).

As shown in the picture, we have a line that represents time passing by: it can be shown in seconds, minutes, hours, days, months or years, according to the shock occurred.

time →

Above this line the sympathetic nervous system - also called orthosympathetic - is shown. (see Appendix)

Sympathicotonia

t →

Under the timeline the parasympathetic nervous system is shown.

t →

Vagotonia

Usually we are in a status of normotonia.

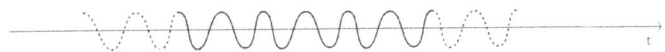

That is to say we physiologically fluctuate from a sympathetic nervous system activation to the parasympathetic nervous system activation: it is the day-night rhythm and the rest-activity rhythm.

During this normotonia -this is quite normal- an acute, unexpected, sudden, dramatic event may occur, which catches me off-guard and I live it as a state of isolation.

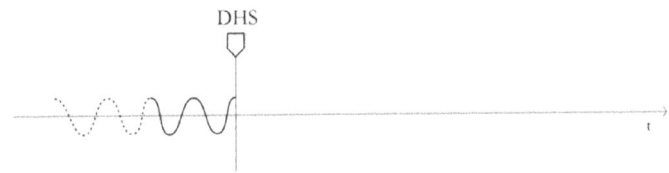

This event (DHS) represents the beginning of a cascade of immediate modifications that will occur simultaneously and instantly at three levels: at a psychic level I will have the memory of the biological conflict (DHS), at brain level, there will be an activation of the cerebral areas (HH-Hamer Focus) that are connected to the event experienced, while at an organ or bowel level, there will be some functional and structural modifications still connected to the event.

The DHS is a biological and not a psychological event.

The living organism should react in an optimal way and straight away to this event, as there is a risk for its safety, its own existence or the existence of the group to which it belongs.

2ʳᵈ Biological Law of Nature

All Special Programs with the Biological Sense(SBS) consist of two phases, provided that you get to the solution of the conflict.

The 2ⁿᵈ Biological Law describes the Significant Biological Special Programs of Nature (SBS) : the biphasic state of the sympaticotonia/parasympaticotonia following the biological conflict (DHS) experienced by the individual at a given moment and it is marked by a series of specific events:

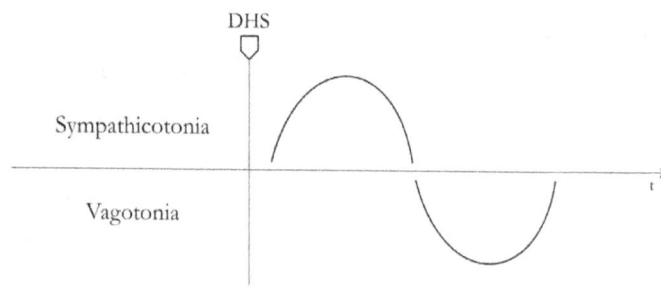

Since DHS has occurred, following a fully meaningful logic from a biological point of view, one can see an activation of the orthosympathetic nervous system: this activation is absolutely optimal to allow the individual to react to that sudden, unexpected event that has caught him off-guard.

The activation of the ortosympathetic system will last until the initial conflict is resolved (DHS). This status of sympathicotonia can be more or less intense (shock mass) depending on the type of conflict experienced. Throughout the sympaticotonia status there will be physic and psychic signs that will show one is in a Conflict Active phase (CA):

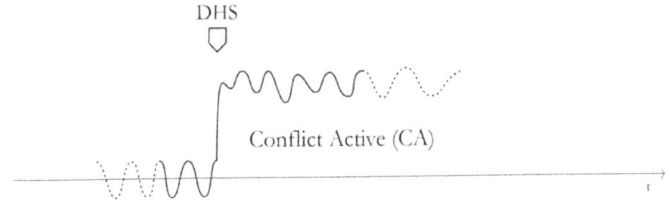

On a psyche level, the person will continue to think about what has happened (obsessive thought), day and night (if it has been particularly intense): this is due to the activation of the sympathethic nervous system.

On a vegetative level, the person will have cold hands and feet, cold skin, lack of appetite, weight loss, insomnia with awakenings between 1 and 3 am and hyperactivity; all this is due to the constant stimulation of the sympathethic nervous system.

On a cerebral level, there will be the formation of the so called Hamer Foci (HH) in specific areas related to the experienced conflict and the corresponding organ. These can be seen during a CAT/CT scan (computerized axial tomography) without contrast.

On an organic level, there will be a structural and functional modification, depending on the embryological origin of the tissue being stimulated by the sympathetic system (3rd Biological Law). During the Active Conflict phase, there are no symptoms (with notably rare exceptions).

This sympathicotonia status following the DHS allows the individual to be able to resolve the conflict in good time (days, weeks or months) and if it happens, this is called Conflictolysis (CL):

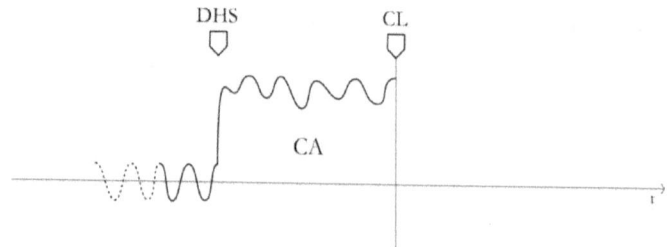

Conflictolysis marks the transition to a second phase, opposite to the first, where there is an activation of the parasympathethic nervous system or vagotonia.

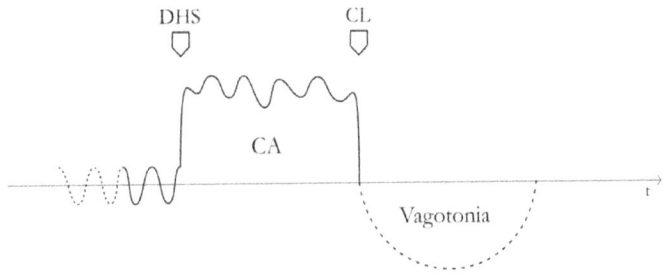

This second vagotonic phase is composed of a phase called A (PCL-A Post-Conflictolysis A), a sympathicotonic phase or peak (Epileptoid Crisis, CE) and a phase B (PCL-B or Post-Conflictolysis B). The duration of this phase is related to the duration of the Conflict Active phase:

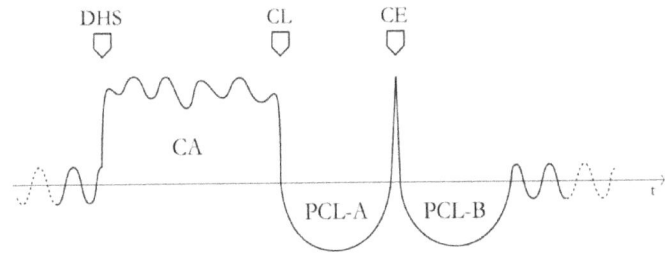

"Just to allow the reader to understand the performance of the 2nd Biological Law discovered by Dr.Hamer, I have reproduced here the biphasic curve chart which partly calls to mind the original by Dr.Hamer as reported in Bibliography."

Throughout the vagotonic status, I will have physic and psychic symptoms that will indicate that I am in a PCL (Post-Conflictolysis) status, also called Healing Phase.

On a psyche level, one will no longer think of the event occurred, as this is now settled and remote, and one will be very calm.

On a vegetative level, one will have: warm hands and feet, fatigue.

On a cerebral level, the so-called Hamer Focus (HF) will show a different conformation of the specific areas related to the experienced conflict and the corresponding organ. These can be seen during a CAT scan (computerized axial tomography) without contrast.

On an organic level, there will be a structural and functional modification,it being the opposite of the sympathicotonic phase one (3rd Biological Law). At this stage, signs and physical symptoms appear, which are precisely related to the DHS suffered previously.

3rd Biological Law of Nature

The ontogenetically conditioned system of the Significant Biological Special Programs of Nature (SBS)

Each tissue originally stems from one of the three embryonic germ layers called: Endoderm, Mesoderm (old and new), Ectoderm (see Appendix); every single tissue derived from a specific embryonic germ layer is subject to a stimulation of the autonomic nervous system (sympathicotonia-parasympathicotonia) and can be subject to one of the four different structural and functional alterations:

- tissue increase (proliferation)

- tissue reduction (necrosis, ulceration)

- increased tissue function (hyperfunction)

- reduced tissue function (hypofunction)

All the tissues that are derived from Endoderm, in the sympathicotonic phase (CA) will have a tissue and function increase, while in the parasympaticotonic phase (PCL) they will have a loss of function and tissue:

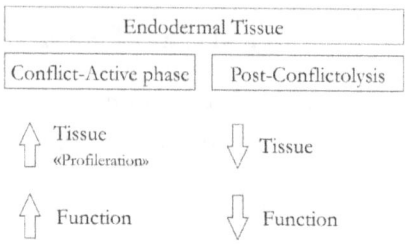

All the tissues that derive from Old Mesoderm, in the sympathicotonic phase (CA) will show a loss of tissue and function, while in the parasympathicotonic phase (PCL)they will show an increase of function and tissue:

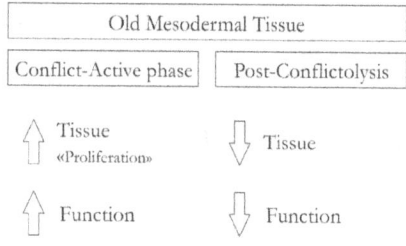

All the tissues deriving from New Mesoderm, in the sympathicotonic phase (CA) will have a loss of tissue and function, while in the parasympathicotonic phase (PCL) they will have an increase of function and tissue:

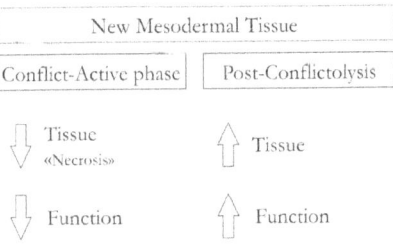

All the tissues that come from Ectoderm, in the sympathicotonic phase (CA) face a loss of tissue and function, while in the parasympathicotonic phase (PCL) they face an increase of function and tissue:

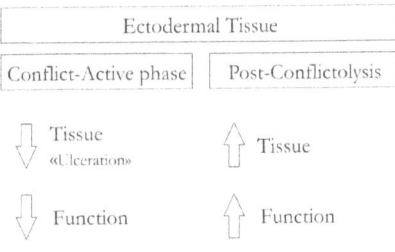

4th Biological Law of Nature

The genetically determined microbial system in the History of Evolution.

Fungi, bacteria and viruses are actively involved in the 2nd phase of the bi-phasic curve (PCL), optimizing the resolution phase.

Endodermal Tissue	Mesodermal Tissue	Ectodermal Tissue
Fungi, Mycobacteria		
	Bacteria	
		Virus

The **Fungi and Mycobacteria** (TBC) participate in the reduction of the tissue deriving from Endoderm that in the active phase (CA) was increased or they do a caseification only during the post-conflict phase. The mycobacteria can also be found in some tissues derived from Old Mesoderm.

The **Bacteria** that derive from Mesoderm proliferate in the active phase (CA) and optimize the tissue healing phase (PCL)

The **Viruses** are in the tissues that derive from Ectoderm in PCL phase and optimize the reconstruction process, restoring the structure.

5th Biological Law of Nature

The quintessence

The 5th biological law reminds us that the Significant Biological Special Programs of Nature (SBS) activated with a DHS have a specific biological sense to ensure the survival of the individual or of the group.

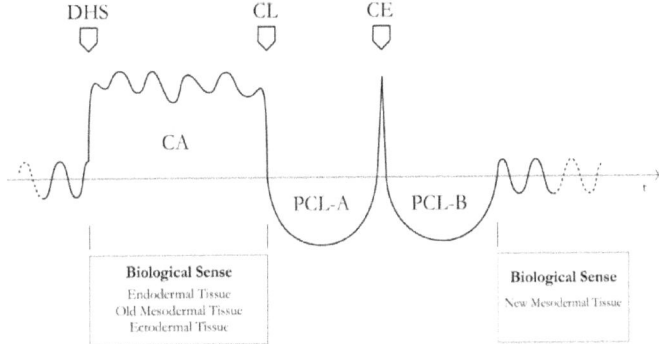

The biological sense is for all tissues in the Active Conflict phase, except for tissues that derive from the New Mesoderm, directed by the White Matter, in which it occurs at the end of the healing phase (normotonia).

2. Biological conflicts

Among all the events that a person experiences, only some will represent a DHS. These are all those conflicts in which the following conditions occur:

- unexpected
- sudden
- acute
- dramatic
- experienced in isolation

They are called Biological Conflicts as the occurring event represents a "biological difficulty" which the individual has to overcome and respond to, in order to ensure its biological integrity, survival or integrity of the group to which it belongs.

The reaction is automatic, immediate, instinctive and not mediated by ego; only these conflicts can be called biological and are the only ones that will allow to start the Significant Special Biological Program (SBS); completely different from those conflicts, in Psychology, in which conflict is a clash between what a person desires and his/her inner/interpersonal needs and this clash doesn't allow the satisfaction of this desire, of the need itself or of the objective related to that desire: these are certainly inconveniences for the individual, but will not be capable of causing the activation of a Significant Biological Special Program.

The biological conflicts that can issue a DHS, are the following:

- "Morsel" conflicts
- "Attack" conflicts *(or fear of being attacked)*
- "Self-devaluation" conflicts
- "Territory and separation" conflicts

Only these conflicts and only if experienced as DHS by the individual (unexpected, sudden, dramatic and lived in isolation) will cause functional and tissue alterations as a significant answer, following the trend of the biphasic curve and the 3rd Biological Law.

Conflicts and the Significant Biological Special Program (SBS) that are produced, allow us both as individuals and as a species to survive in worst-case scenarios and in less dramatic cases to react to the unexpected occurred event.

"Morsel" conflict

These conflicts are related to the survival of the individual, of his species and the maintenance of vital functions: eating, digesting, assimilating, eliminating, evacuating, breathing, hearing and reproduction.

The morsel conflict, with all its variants, involves all the tissues that derive from Endoderm, that is to say from that embryonic germ layer directly involved in preserving the body's vital functions; these are the tissues:

- Oral Submucosa
- Palate
- Parotid Glands
- Sublingual Salivary Glands
- Tonsils
- Naso-Pharynx
- Lacrimal glands
- Iris
- Thyroid Gland
- Neurohypophysis
- Middle ear

- Eustachian tube
- Esophagus *(lower third only)*
- Lung alveoli
- Stomach *(greater curvature only)*
- Duodenum *(except for duodenal bulb)*
- Liver parenchyma *(no bile ducts nor cholecyst)*
- Pancreas parenchyma *(except for pancreatic ducts and Langerhans islets)*
- Small and Large Intestine *(Colon)*
- Tongue
- Sigmoid and Rectum *(upper third)*
- Bladder
- Kidney Collecting Tubules
- Prostate
- Uterus and Fallopian Tubes
- Bartholin's glands
- Smegma glands
- Inner navel
- Nuclei of the Acoustic Nerves

The morsel, which is essential for the survival of the individual, is associated to food as well as air morsel (lung alveoli), light morsel (eye, enteroidea), sound morsel (middle ear), water morsel (kidney collecting tubules).

The emotional contents of the morsel conflicts related to man are, to name just a few:

- conflict of "not being able to digest a morsel"

- conflict of "not being able to swallow a morsel"
- death-fright conflict
- conflict of "inability to catch a morsel"
- …

For a detailed study of conflicts relating to DHS , may the reader view the Scientific Table of Germanic New Medicine® (Ed.Amici di Dirk).

"Attack" Conflicts (or fear of being attacked)

These conflicts are related to feeling attacked by everything surrounding the individual, feeling one's own integrity attacked.

The conflict of feeling attacked, with all its variants, involves all tissues that derive from Old Mesoderm, the embryonic germ layer directly concerned with the protection of the individual; these are the tissues:

- **Corium Skin** *(derma)*
- Breast Glands (milk producing glands) *(except for ducts)*
- Pericardium *(sac containing the heart)*
- Pleura *(lining of the lungs)*
- Peritoneum *(membrane lining of the abdominal cavity and abdominal organs)*
- Greater Omentum

The emotional contents of Attack conflicts (or fear of being attacked) related to man are, to name just a few:

- Conflict of rejecting contact
- Conflict of attack to one's integrity
- Conflict of personal disfigurement
- Conflict of attack against one's heart
- ...

Conflict of "self-devaluation"

These conflicts are related to feeling devaluated, fear of failing, not feeling adequate, not being good at doing something, not being up to scratch.

The self-devaluation conflict, with all its variables, involves all the tissues that derive from New Mesoderm, that is to say that embryonic germ layer involved in the individual's growth and strengthening of the group; these are the derived tissues:

- Bones (including tooth dentin)
- Cartilage
- Tendons and Ligaments
- Connective tissue
- Fat tissue
- Lymphatic system (Lymph vessels & Lymphnodes)
- Blood vessels (except coronary vessels)
- Muscles (striated musculature)

- Myocardium (80% striated heartmuscle)
- Kidney Parenchyma
- Adrenal cortex
- Spleen
- Ovaries
- Testicles

The emotional contents of the devaluation conflicts related to the individual are, to name just a few:

- Conflict of intellectual devaluation
- Conflict of not being adequate
- Conflict of incapability to escape a situation
- Conflict of feeling left outside a situation
- Conflict of having lost someone
- Conflict of being tied to a ball and chain
- …

"Territory and separation" conflicts

These conflicts are related to the group to which one belongs, to the territory and separation. The territorial conflict (fight and separation), with all its variants, involves all tissues that stem from Ectoderm, that is to say that embryonic germ layer directly connected to territorial fight and separation. These are the tissues stemming from the ectoderm:

- **Epidermis** *(skin)*

- Periosteum *(skin that covers the bones)*
- Mouth *(upper mucosa)*, incl. palate, gums, tongue, lining of salivary gland ducts
- Nasal and sinuses membrane
- Inner ear
- Lens, cornea, conjunctiva, retina, and vitreous body of the eyes
- Teeth enamel
- Lining of the milk ducts
- Lining of the thyroid gland ducts and of pharyngeal ducts
- Lining of the heart vessels *(coronary arteries and coronary veins)*
- Esophagus *(upper 2/3)*
- Laryngeal mucosa and Bronchial mucosa
- Stomach lining *(small curvature)*
- Lining of the bile ducts and gall bladder, and of pancreatic ducts
- Cervix and vagina
- Lining of renal pelvis, bladder, ureter, and urethra
- Lining of the rectum *(lower part)*
- Nerve cells of the Central Nervous System

The emotional contents of territorial conflicts related to man are, to name just a few :

- Territorial conflict
- Territorial threatening conflict
- Territorial anger conflict

- Conflict of inability of marking the territory
- Separation conflict
- Conflict of having no right to bite

For a detailed study of conflicts relating to DHS may the reader refer to the Scientific Table of Germanic New Medicine® (Ed. Amici di Dirk).

3. The "Conflict Active" phase

The DHS that occurred marks the beginning of the Significant Biologic Special program of Nature. The sympathethic nervous system will be activated to bring a response to the event, which occurred so suddenly and unexpectedly, in order to solve it as soon as possible: this phase is called Conflict Active (CA).

The individual in a Conflict Active phase will continue to mull all day long over that event that occurred so unexpectedly and, if this event has been very intense, the person will think about it also during the night and wake up between 1 and 3 am. On a somatic level,the individual will have very cold hands and feet, lack of appetite, hyperactivity, mild fatigue.

During the Conflict Active phase, the individual is fine and has no symptoms that can worry him, all his physical and mental energies are directed to solve his problem (DHS). Other smaller problems are momentarily put aside and, in any case, they are not a priority at this time.

In this phase, depending on the type of conflict (DHS) experienced by the individual, the tissues begin to "respond" to the sympathicotonia status but there are no symptoms:

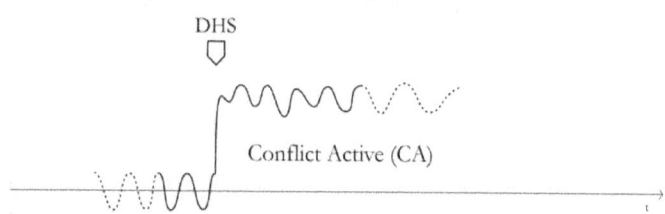

If DHS is related to a morsel conflict corresponding to a tissue that derives from Endoderm, in the Conflict Active phase, the tissue will increase (proliferation) and its related function will increase as well:

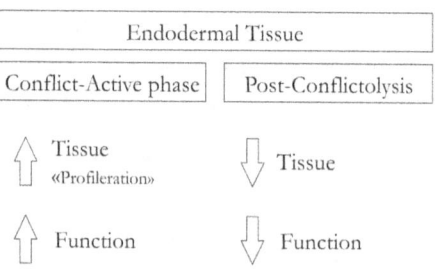

If DHS is related to an attack conflict corresponding to a tissue that derives from Old Mesoderm, in the Conflict Active phase, the tissue will increase and its related function will increase as well:

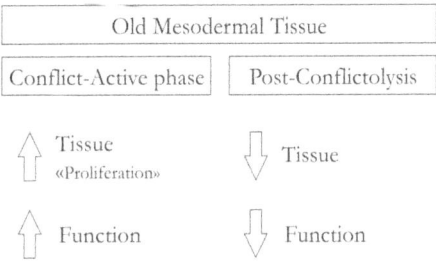

If DHS is related to a self-devaluation conflict corresponding to a tissue that derives from New Mesoderm, in the Conflict Active phase, the tissue will be reduced and so will its related function:

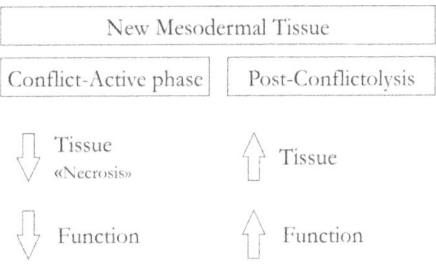

If DHS is related to a territorial conflict corresponding to a tissue that comes from Endoderm, in the Conflict Active phase, the tissue will be reduced (ulceration) and so will its function:

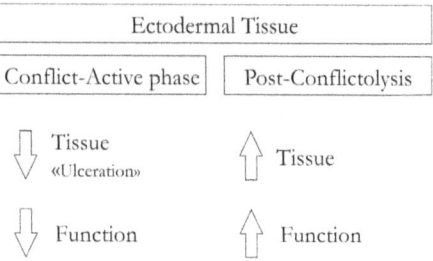

The biological sense (5th Biological Law) for all conflicts that derive from Endoderm, from Old Mesoderm and Ectoderm is in the Conflict Active phase:

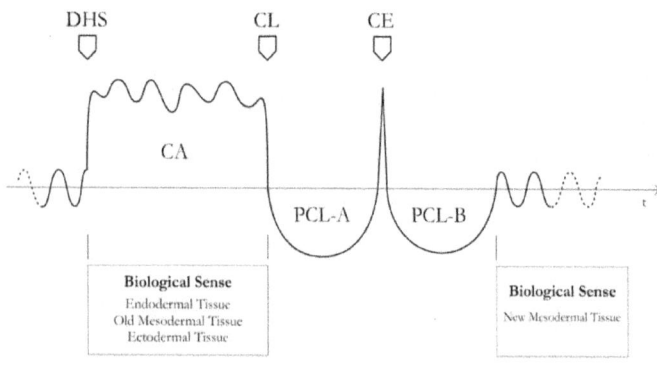

4. Conflictolysis

Conflictolysis occurs when, thanks to the state of sympathicotonia, I have been in, I am able to resolve the conflict (DHS). The resolution of the conflict can happen in different ways, more or less depending on the individual; one can manage to finally get away from what has happened, one can deal with the situation or, it may occur, circumstances spontaneously evolve in a better direction even without one's direct intervention:

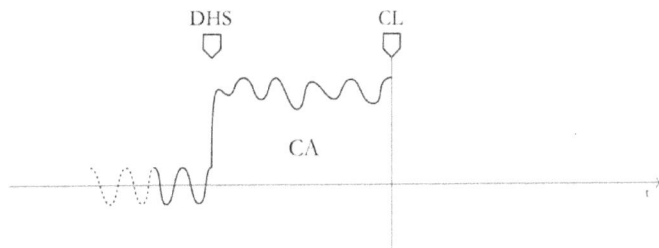

Conflictolysis is an event that allows the resolution of a biological conflict, has a positive connotation, it represents a relief, a solution.

After Conflictolysis, a phase change occurs; from a status of ortosympathicotonia, a parasympathicotonia or vagotonic phase will appear and this is called Post-Conflictolysis phase of resolution.

5. Post-Conflictolysis Phase

The Healing phase - Post Conflictolysis (PCL) represents the second phase of the biphasic curve; the autonomic nervous system switches from activation of the sympathetic to an activation of the parasympathetic:

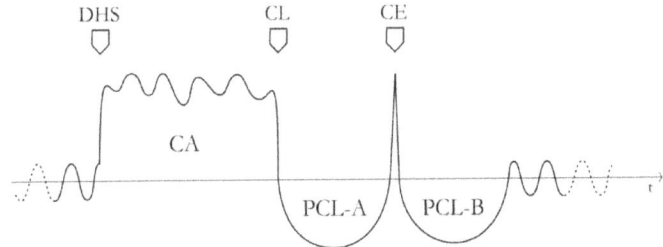

In this vagotonic phase, the individual will be tired and will sleep longer than usual if possible, he will no longer think of his problem because it is finally solved and at a somatic level he will have warm hands, feet and skin and he will see signs and symptoms that will prompt him to a medical consultation to give a name to his "disease".

The symptoms that occur in this phase are related to the type of DHS occurred earlier and which started the Significant Biological Special program: a cold, bronchitis, vitiligo, dermatitis, gastritis, hepatitis, cystitis, psoriasis, pleurisy, conjunctivitis, myopia, low back pain, rhinitis, headache, arthritis... and all the so-called "diseases" that have a precise and unique correspondence with a biological conflict (DHS)

In this second phase called vagotonic, the tissues begin to respond to the parasympathicotonic phase (3rd Biological Law):

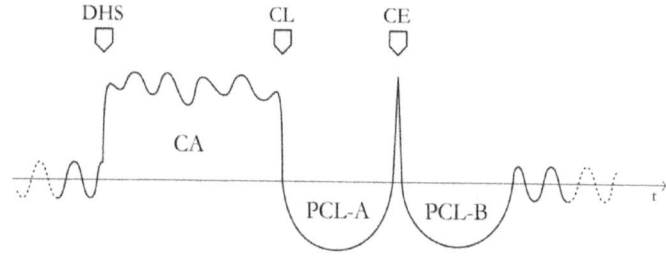

If DHS is related to a morsel conflict, that corresponds to any tissue that derives from Endoderm in resolution, the tissue and its function will be reduced:

| Endodermal Tissue |
| Conflict-Active phase | Post-Conflictolysis |

Tissue «Profileration» ↑ | Tissue ↓
Function ↑ | Function ↓

If DHS is related to a attack conflict, that corresponds to any tissue that derives from Old Mesoderm in resolution, the tissue and its function will be reduced:

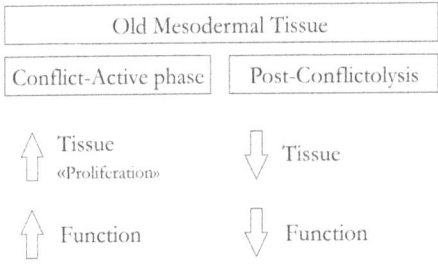

| Old Mesodermal Tissue |
| Conflict-Active phase | Post-Conflictolysis |

Tissue «Proliferation» ↑ | Tissue ↓
Function ↑ | Function ↓

If DHS is related to a devaluation conflict, corresponding to any tissue deriving from the New Mesoderm in resolution, the tissue and its function will end this phase with a surplus of tissue:

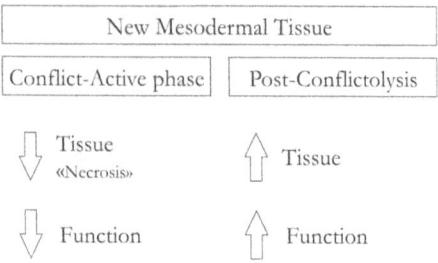

If DHS is related to a territorial conflict, that corresponds to any tissue that derives from Ectoderm in resolution, the tissue and its function will be replenished:

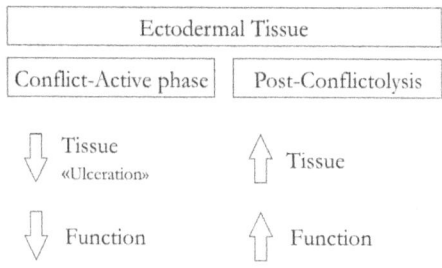

As you can see in this picture, the vagotonic resolution phase is composed by three curves:

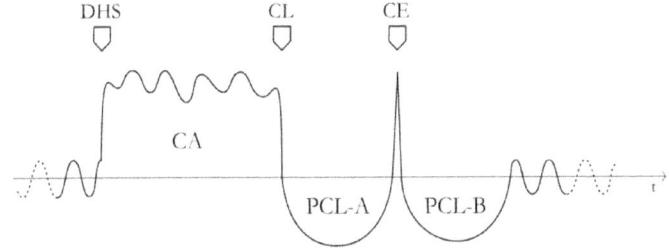

The PCL A (Post-Conflictolysis phase A) is the first parasympathicotonic in which one or more symptoms appear. Analysing a single biphasic curve and without conflict relapses, the temporal duration of this phase is exactly half the duration of the Conflict Active phase but with a maximum duration of 3 weeks (e.g.):

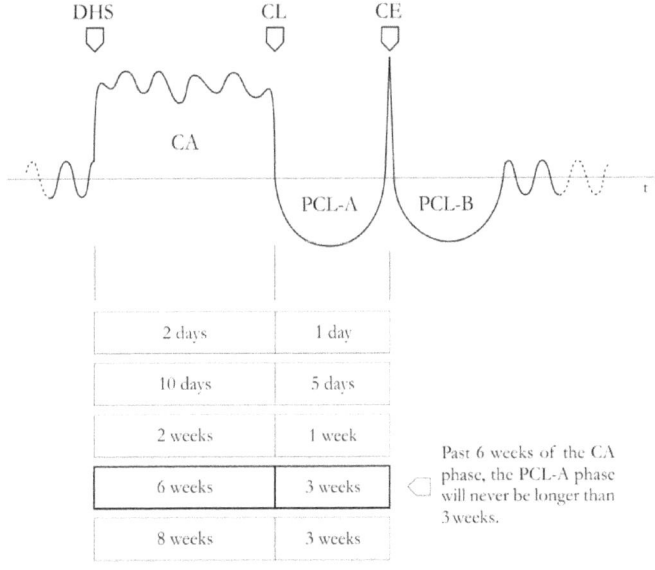

2 days	1 day
10 days	5 days
2 weeks	1 week
6 weeks	3 weeks
8 weeks	3 weeks

Past 6 weeks of the CA phase, the PCL-A phase will never be longer than 3 weeks.

If the CA phase lasted two weeks, the PCL A phase has a duration of one week. Past 6 weeks of the CA phase, the PCL A phase will never be longer than 3 weeks).

After the PCL A phase, a sympathicotonic peak is shown, which is called EPILEPTOID CRISIS (EPI-CRISIS) (CE) (If DHS is motorial, it will be called Epileptic crisis). This sympathicotonic peak occurs in the middle of the healing phase and its function is to reduce the brain edema at the HH level : it will be associated to very intense and acute symptoms called renal colic, biliary colic, intestinal colic, panic attack (and more) but it will always be in relation to the emotional content of the initial DHS.

Biologically, the epi-crysis has a duration that can range from 10 -20 seconds to 4 hours:

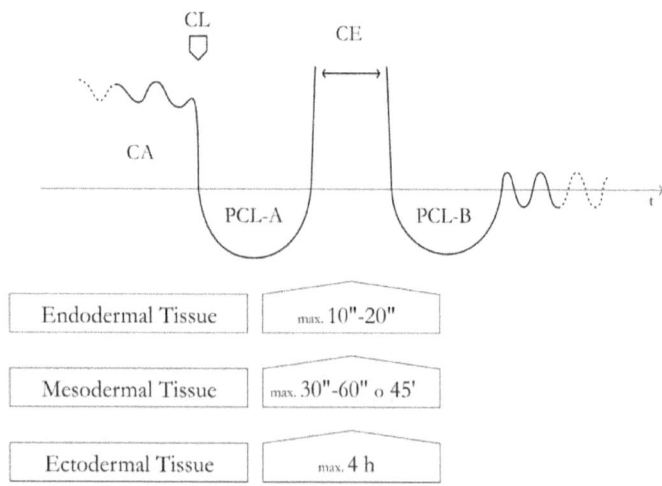

Endodermal Tissue	max. 10"-20"
Mesodermal Tissue	max. 30"-60" o 45'
Ectodermal Tissue	max. 4 h

The duration of the Epi-crysis, it often happens, can exceed maximum if it enters a "hanging" phase.

At the end of the Epileptoid crisis a vagotonic phase will recur, called PCL B, with less intense symptoms, which will mark the end of the Significant Biological special Program of Nature before getting back to normotonia:

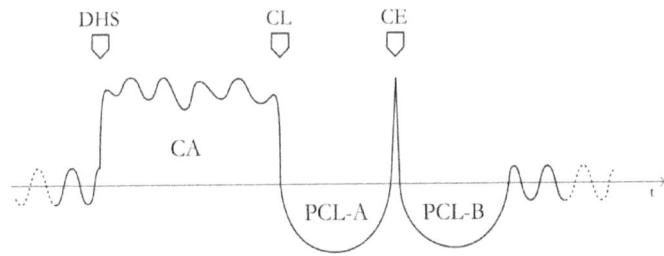

During the Post-Conflictolysis phase, besides having the specific symptoms determined by the DHS and the type of tissue involved, one may also run a temperature of varying degrees, depending on the embryonic derivation of tissue:

body temperature   37°C   38°C   39°C   40°C

Endodermal Tissue		
Mesodermal Tissue		
Ectodermal Tissue		

The biological sense (5ᵗʰ Biological Law) for tissues that derive from the new Mesoderm comes at the end of the biphasic curve, when normotonia is restored:

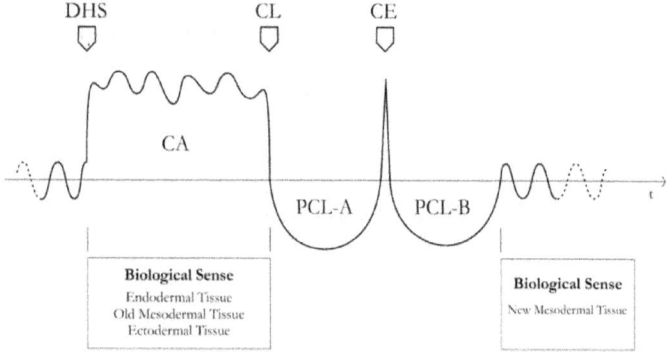

6. Laterality

It is fundamental to know whether you are right- or left-handed to understand how the individual functions.

Of all the tests that can be done to determine whether you are right-handed or left-handed, Dr. Hamer was able to verify that the only suitable one to establish the exact laterality is the one of applause.

By applauding like in a theater, the hand that beats above gives dominance: the right-handed individual will hit his right hand over the left while the left-handed will hit his left hand over the right one.

In right-handed people, both male and female, the non-dominant side, the left one ,is related to the nest, to their mother and their children or animals.The right side applies to all other figures (father, husband, lover, friend, friends, girl-friends, employer, in-laws ...):

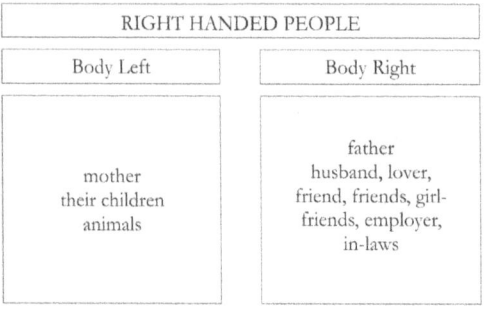

In left-handed people, both male and female, the non-dominant side, the right one, is in relation to their mother and their children, or animals, while the dominant regards all other persons:

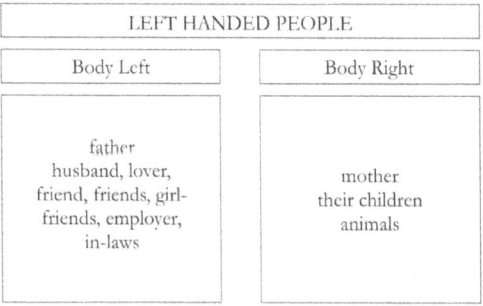

The rule of laterality applies only to tissues that derive from Mesoderm and Ectoderm.

7. Hanging healings

When a DHS occurs, the individual goes from a Conflict Active phase (CA) to a Conflictolysis and then a vagotonic Post-Conflictolysis phase starts and will return, with its biologic time, to a normotonia.

We call it "hanging healing" when the individual, instead of progressing to the biphasic curve, as described, will keep going from one vagotonic phase(PCL) to a sympathicotonic one (CA), not necessarily returning to normotonia.

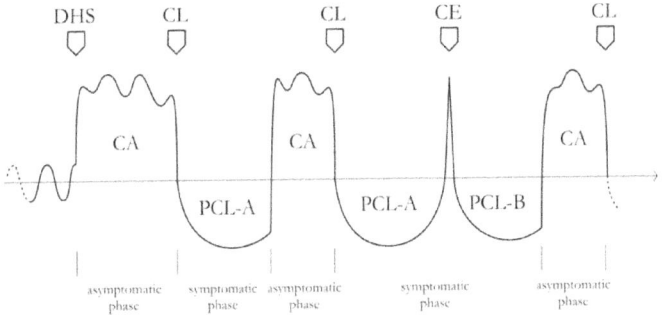

This pattern is due to the fact that, when one is in a vagotonic phase of CA, the event occurs again bringing one back into a Conflict Active phase. This trend can last long, even for months.

As to symptoms, they will show in a vagotonic phase (PCL) and then one will experience a fading or disappearance of symptoms in the sympathycotonic phase (CA).

8. Conflict Relapses or "Tracks"

At the exact time DHS occurs, our nervous system records not only the conflict that will trigger the Significant Biologic Special Program but also all those "signals" that accompanied the DHS.

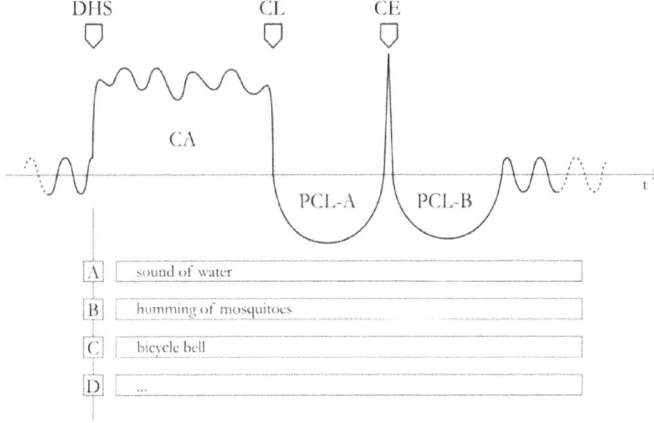

If a DHS of any kind occurs while I am walking on a riverside, in addition to the DHS I will fix a series of "signs", for example, the sound of water, the humming of mosquitoes , the local temperature, the bicycle bell and so on.

These "signals" in future, if reappearing all together or isolated from one another, will reactivate the original biphasic curve related to the event previously experienced years before; if this occurs, as an effect, I will see symptoms showing in relation to the curve.

This mode, from a biological point of view, is optimal because it is a "warning signal" to prevent one from bumping into such a peculiar situation that has already occurred.

9. Refugee Conflict

Whenever one experiences DHS, a new Biological Program(SBS) begins, so if one has different DHS at the same time, one will have different bi-phasic curves, some in an active phase and some in resolution:

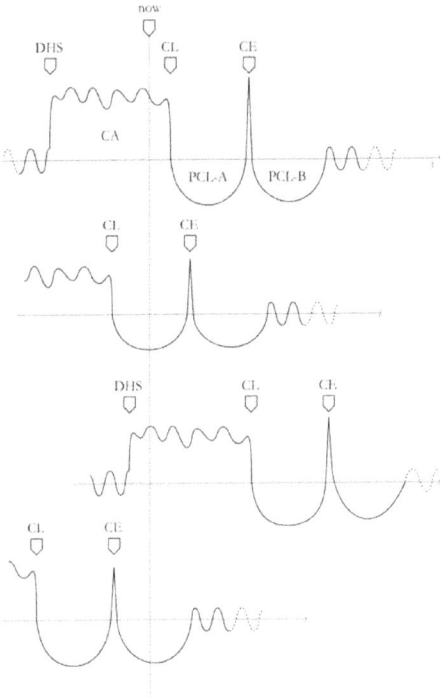

This means that, in a given moment, one will be in CA for one or more DHS, in PCL-A for one or more DHS and in PCL-B for one or more other DHS.

So: for the conflicts I will be having in CA, I will show no symptoms but I will not sleep at night and will feel anxiety.

Instead, I will have a particularly annoying symptom about the conflict in the PCL A phase and a different symptom for the PCL B phase of the DHS that I am living, but at least for this latter conflict in the solution phase I am much calmer and the worst is over.

Among all the biological conflicts we are having, there is a very important and essential one, for its practical implications that can increase, if it is active, the symptomatic manifestation of the parasympatheticotonic curve (PCL-A and B) as well as of any biphasic curve related to an active SBS.

This is the refugee conflict, a program of water retention, related to the system of kidney collecting tubules (derivating from Endoderm) that in the Conflict Active phase, increase their function:

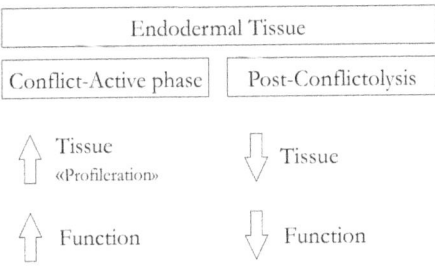

During the sympathicotonic phase of the kidney collecting tubules:

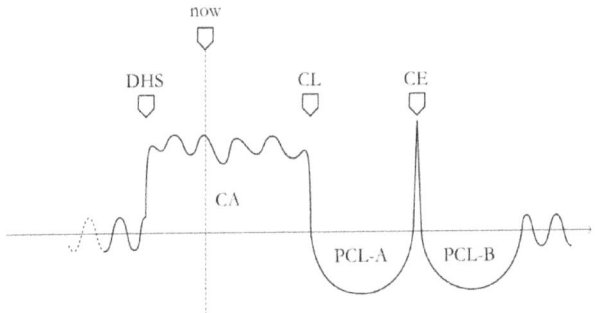

I will experience systemic water retention (the whole body will feel bloated): I will feel bloated, not necessarily with other symptoms, but if in addition to the SBS of collecting tubules(active refugee conflict) I also have another SBS in a solution A phase (PCL-A), the symptoms of this conflict will increase exponentially.

The result will be a local edema of the 2nd curve plus global edema (CA of the kidney collecting tubules) of the 1st curve and this will cause more serious symptoms (local edema + global edema = more pain or symptom):

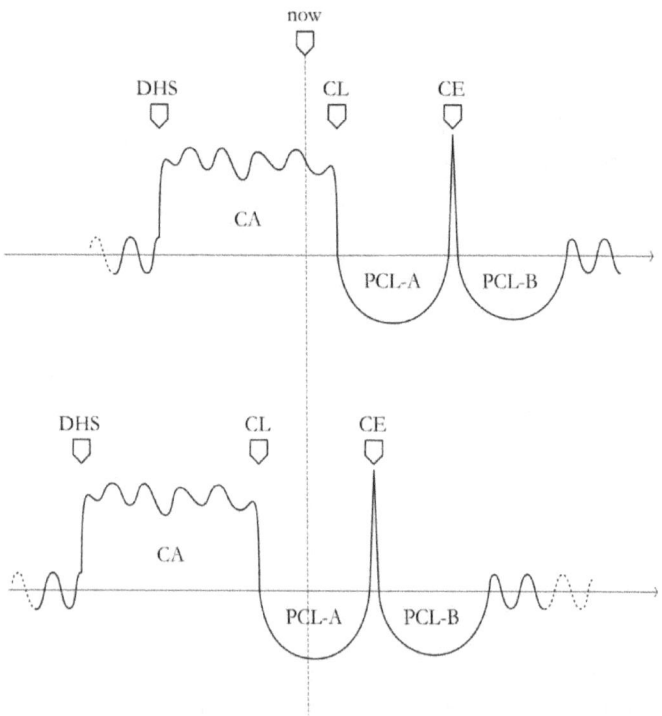

A single healing curve (PCL) gives an ache or a symptom that can reach 2-3 in a range from 1 to 10. Together with an active refugee conflict, the ache goes up to 9-10.

10. The skin

In order to better understand the conflicts and, above all, the somatic manifestations of the dermatological diseases in the light of Dr. Hamer's discoveries, it is essential to define:

- the embryological derivation of the affected tissues

- tissues involved in the conflicts of the skin

- which conflicts are related to the skin

- 3rd - 4th - 5th Biological Law

Although the skin is composed of several layers of cells, overlaid with precise functions, it is possible to distinguish basically two main layers, epidermis and derma:

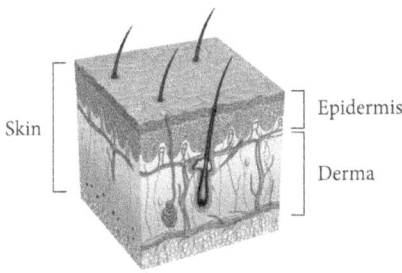

Skin

Epidermis

Derma

From embryology we know that:

- From the Ectoderm derive cells that make up the epidermis and the hair follicle with its hair.
- From the Ancient Mesoderm derive cells that make up the derma, the sebaceous and sweat glands.

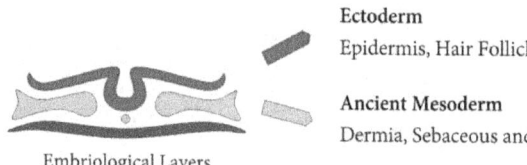

Ectoderm
Epidermis, Hair Follicle, Hair

Ancient Mesoderm
Dermia, Sebaceous and Sweat Glands

Embriological Layers

From Dr. Hamer's discoveries we know that:

- The epidermis and the hair follicle "respond" to the conflicts of "separation and loss" .
- The derma, the sebaceous and sweat glands "respond" to the conflict "of feeling attacked", assaulted, conflicts incident to dirtiness.

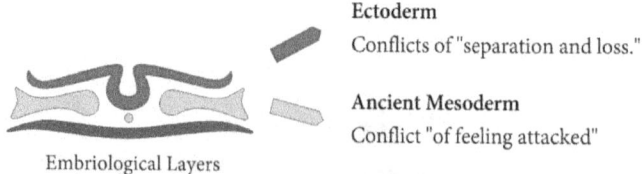

Ectoderm
Conflicts of "separation and loss."

Ancient Mesoderm
Conflict "of feeling attacked"

Embriological Layers

Through the 3rd Biological Law we know the behavior of the tissue in relation to autonomic nervous stimulation:

- The epidermis and its appendages of ectodermic origin leads in sympathicotonia to a reduction of function and tissue, while in para-sympathicotonia leads to a restoration of function and tissue, in normotonia it leads to a reactivation of the normal functionality:

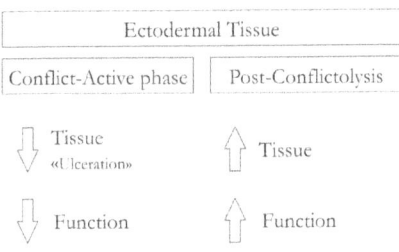

- The derma and its appendages of ancient mesodermal origin, in sympathicotonia leads to an increase of function and tissue (proliferation), while in para-sympathicotonia leads to a function and tissue reduction, in normotonia it remains more or less an excess of tissue:

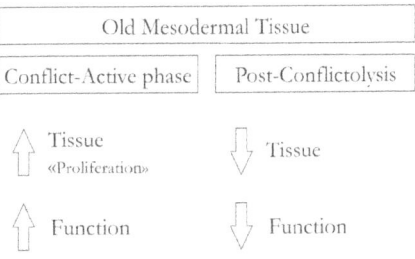

Regarding the 4th Biological Law we know that:

- The viruses optimize the phase of repair (PCL) of the tissues derived from the Ectoderm.
- Fungi optimize the phase of repair (PCL) of the tissues derived from the ancient mesoderm.

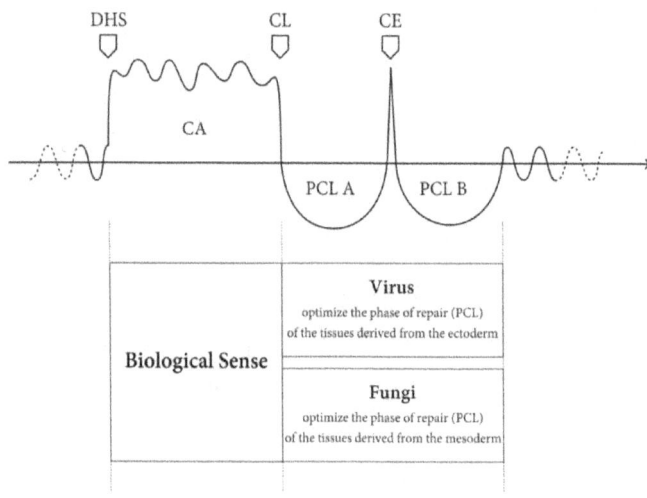

As for the 5th Biological Law, which defines the biological sense, it is for both tissues in sympathicotonia (CA).

Prior to observe and explain the so-called "dermatological pathologies", we can make a handy summary about the morphology of the "cutaneous lesions" and their symptomatic manifestation. Broadly, on a cutaneous level, we can always describe the same signs which may show different shades depending on the intensity of the conflict (conflicting mass), on relapses and each one will be assigned with a specific name (vitiligo, psoriasis, labial herpes, acne ...).

Epidermis

The epidermis "responds" to the Conflicts of separation and, according to CA (Active Conflict) or PCL (Post-Conflict Solution), we will have several changes only in relation to the autonomic nervous activation:

Dry Skin

Dry skin indicates the active conflict phase (CA) in a separation conflict.

Skin from rose-coloured to reddened

It indicates a parasympathicotonic phase (PCLA-PCLB), that is to say of resolution in a conflict of separation.

Cutaneous hypopigmentation

Sympathicotonic phase of the epidermis (CA).

Skin that flakes off

Parasympaticotonic phase (PCLB) of the epidermis.

Itch

Epileptic crisis (EC) of a conflict of separation.

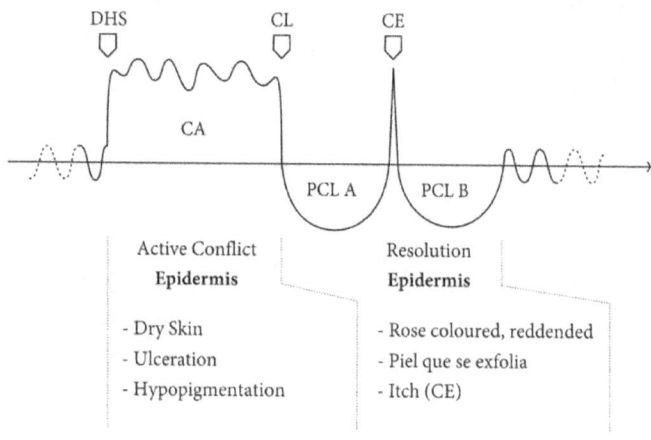

Ulceration

Separation conflict with several relapses. Ulceration appears after the first relapse.

Sweat

Ipersweating (CA) of the sweat glands without odor.

The derma

The derma "responds" to the Conflicts of protection, or "feeling attacked", assaulted, to the conflicts of dirtiness or of loss of physical integrity and, according to being in CA or PCL phase, we will have several modifications only in relation to the autonomic nervous activation:

Thickening of the derma

if the thickening is melanotic (CA) at a level/layer of the derma.

if the thickening is amelanotic (CA) at a deeper level/layer relative to the derma.

Cutaneous Hypopigmentation

Sympathicotonic phase of the derma (CA).

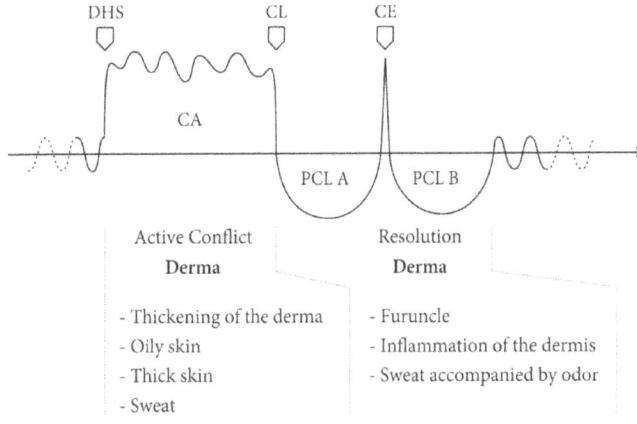

Furuncle

Indicates a parasympathicotonic phase (PCL) of repair.

Oily skin

Sympathicotonia (CA) of the sebaceous glands with numerous relapses.

Thick skin

Sympathicotonia (CA) of the derma with many relapses.

Sweat

Sympathicotonic phase of the sweat glands (CA and CE).

Sweat accompanied by odor

Parasympathicotonic phase of the sweat glands (PCL) and participating reduction due to skin fungi.

11. The dermatological diseases

Once understood the 5 Biological Laws and its practical developments, let us observe certain diseases.

It is important to underline that the areas where the "injuries" appear may be in relation to:

- laterality (right-handedness or left-handedness)

for example, a Labial Herpes on the left side of lips, in a right-hander, will be in relation to a separation conflict from his/her mother or his/her children

- at the local area of the conflict

for example, if I receive a direct attack in a specific area of the body, e.g. because of a stab wound, I will develop a keloid.

Acne Vulgaris

It is the Conflict of "feeling attacked" interpreted as "to like or not to like" typical, but not exclusive, of the pubertal age. To this last one, it may be concomitant a conflict of aesthetic local devaluation.

The sympathicotonic phase goes unnoticed, but during the para-sympaticotonic phase (PCL), under the action of bacteria, small abscesses occur with necrosis and reduction.

The symptomatic phase will produce the beginning of a vicious cycle that will generate several relapses.

Angiomas

Conflicts of separation with devaluation with continuous relapses. The lesion occurs exactly where we have suffered the conflict of separation / depreciation according to the conflicts somatic map in relation to the bones, muscles (Book: The 5 Biological Laws: Bones, Muscles and Joints)

Alopecia , Alopecia Areata

Conflict of intense separation from those who caress or caressed our head. The morphology of alopecia is always related to the type of contact we experienced. During the CA you have hair loss, while in vagotonia (PCL) you have regrowth only if the conflict has not been very intense, and if relapses have not occur.

Androgenic Alopecia

Conflict of separation from the father. The father is not present in our life as we would like. Naturally, after many relapses, the progressive loss of hair occur.

If the hair loss is lateral, it is always related to the separation, but from the mother.

Callosity

Conflict of separation - "aggression" by those who interfere to make us change our mind (by those who step on our toes).

Cellulite

Cellulite comes from conflicts of local aesthetics. If the devaluation type is like I don't like my hips, my buttocks or my thighs, I will develop cellulite on these parts and so on. Here it is involved the connective tissue (derived from recent mesoderm) and so the conflict is of devaluation. From the observation of the precise area with the cellulite, you can get more information on additional concurrent conflicts; in the sense that if there is even dry skin, I will have an ongoing conflict of separation (during the CA); if skin shows "holes", it will present the Conflict of Refugee, a state of water retention in the whole body that will aggravate locally the state of cellulite.

Dermatitis, Eczema (neurodermatitis), Urticaria

It may seem a simplistic view but all these are forms of separation conflict in resolution, that is to say in Post-Conflict Solution (PCL):

the skin appears reddened, hot, dilated, index of vagotonic phase which is always further the Conflict Solution (CL). The area of the manifestation can be related to laterality, or to the place where the separation has taken place, this has to be verified only with the involved person. For example, if I have a dermatitis in the inside medial part of my arms, thoughts will be directed towards a separation from the one who I wanted or I embraced; a dermatitis on the neck or on my face, I will look for a separation from the one who kissed me on the neck and gave me kisses on my face ... the symptomatic manifestation, called dermatitis, for example, always occurs only when there is a reconciliation, when you resume contact.

Each manifestation of the "lesion" is always and constantly dependent on the DHS, the conflicting mass (CA), the resolution (CL), the duration of relapses, the location/s of the body where the separation is experienced. When the lesion takes the form of "map", that is detected, it is to indicate that the person is living, in addition to what is described, the Active Refugee. The hives, itch, if it is present, indicates that you are experiencing the Epileptic Crisis.

Dyshidrosis

In Dyshidrosis the interested tissue is the derma of mesodermal origin; therefore the conflict type is "I feel dirtied, assaulted, attacked".

The lesion, the typical yellow bubbles that open on the surface, occurs just where I felt dirtied / attacked. For example, some people wash dishes by hands without using gloves, and this can often be disgusting; or accidentally we touch things, substances from which we feel to have been dirtied, attacked. For cases of dyshidrosis (relapses) that frequently occur, we should try to think about what we are frequently touching that is disgusting.

Genital Herpes

The Genital Herpes is equal to the Labial One, but the connotation is of course sex.

Labial Herpes

What is defined as Labial Herpes is the result of conflicts of separation, not necessarily of sexual type, from the person we want to kiss. The left-right localization is related to the law of laterality (see Chapter 7). For example, if a young right-hander suffered a conflict of separation from his girlfriend, as a consequence of the reconciliation (Conflict Solution), it will occur the lesion on his lip right. Even the affected lip, upper or lower, gives information about the separation type, the former is more related to the kiss, while the latter is more linked to the expression, separation conflict from the one to whom we want to express in the relationship.

There are cases in which the lesion is inside the nose, in this case is a separation linked to smell / scent of a person, laterality is always respected.

Psoriasis

This type of expression is relative to a double conflict of separation in which the component, more superficial and characterized by silvery scales (dry skin), is related to a separation in an Active Conflict (CA), while the underlying component, inflamed reddened skin, is relative to another conflict of separation concerning another person in the post-conflict solution phase (PCL). It may happen that both phases (AC and PCL) are relative to the same person, that is to say I feel separate and suffer, but I accept it, it's ok but it does not go well, everything at the same time. If the psoriasis state lasts for more than three or four weeks, it is because the person is experiencing relapses. The psoriasis' manifestation starts only when the second separation takes place, being able to "work" later respect to the experienced separation. By lightening biologically and not psychologically, one of the two separations, the psoriasis disappears, leaving only one single separation ongoing in the interested area that, according to the situations, it will be dry skin (CA) or reddened skin (PCL).

Nevi

Small conflicts of separation and "feeling attached"

Moles

Small conflicts of separation and "feeling attached"

Pediculosis

Head lice are found only in those subjects who are in the post-conflict solution phase of a conflict of separation. Individuals who do not have active separation program will not be affected.

Skin Fungi

They are the result of conflicts linked to "feeling attacked" with many relapses. The interested area will give more information about the hint of the conflict. For example, people who experience the fungi on the upper part of the back, they are individuals who are living a situation where they constantly feel attacked (from behind), criticized, judged, ridiculed ...

Sweating

It is necessary to distinguish between the physiological sweating (that allows to cool down) and sweating related to a biological conflict of feeling attacked, assailed. Biologically, if you feel attacked, you sweat (sweat glands) because of the fear and, for the duration of the hazard (CA) perspiration is not combined with smell (the "predator" does not hear our smell).

Going into Conflict Solution (CL), since we put secured, especially in the PCLA phase, we stink besides sweat but this is not a problem being the danger past.

From what explained, it is easy to understand why sometimes we have a "bad smell" and so we will able to pay attention to a quarrel, discussion that we have had a few days or hours before. Individuals who continually stink, it is because they feel constantly attacked, criticized, ridiculed in all environments ...

Urticaria, itch

The itch always refers to the epileptic crisis (EC) of a conflict of separation.

Vitiligo

Vitiligo is a brutal separation conflict with an additional connotation of despicable, bad, unpleasant ("disgusting separation").

In Active Conflict there is a tissue reduction that is hypopigmentation and once the Conflict Solution has passed (CL), the tissue attempts to restore pigmentation. In some lesions on the perimeter appears a red thin edge of regrowth; if the conflict has been very intense, it is not visible.

Warts

They are the result of conflicts of separation with constant relapses with the particular characteristic such as: I would like to have a contact, but I do not have, or just the contrary, I do not want the contact, but I am forced to have it so I want / I do not want the contact.

The different localizations such as fingers, the palm of the hand, feet, depend on the type of contact: the feet are in relation to the "ground" where we walk, the hands are linked to touch and manual dexterity, to write, to play ...

Zoster Herpes

Zoster Herpes is due to a very intense conflict of separation and sometimes it is concomitant to a conflict of zonal "dirtiness". In this case, there is also the formation of pustules that, while opening, can release a fetid odor.

Considerations

From what exposed until now, it is possible to verify that the dermatological lesions solely depend on what we have experienced and what we are going on to live in relation to the initial conflict.

Although after a medical diagnosis defining exactly the name of one's skin disease, the lesion does not always remain the same over time, but undergoes phases of remission and exacerbation, the explanation of these changes is to be found exclusively by involving the interested person and investigating his experience.

Looking for conflicts of separation, it is often difficult to make the person remember when the event started. From the biological point of view the reason is logical since, taking place a separation behind which there is always pain and suffering, the memory fails. Trying to remember the event, the temporal space, where the person places the event, can also be wrong even of 2-3 years.

12. Pharmacological Therapies

The drugs interact chemically with the tissues. Basically the cortisone medicines, antifungal and antibacterial medications have a sympathetic property, that is artificially and chemically, they bring the tissue in a state of sympathicotonia (CA), where according to the 2nd Biological Law, we know that we have not any symptoms.

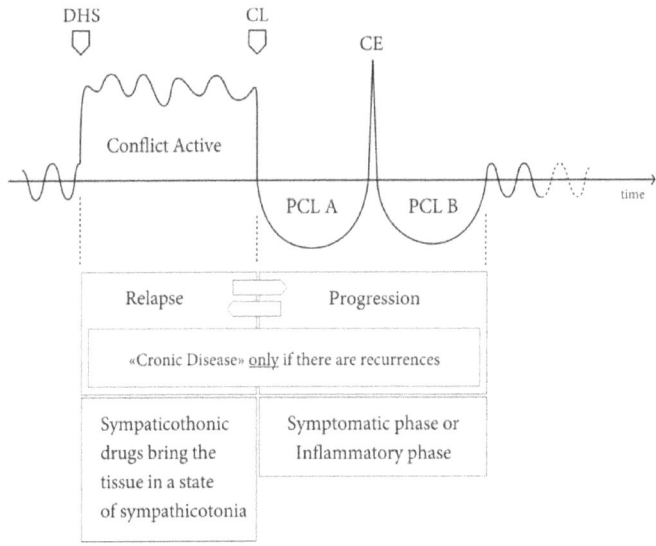

A tissue, for example the skin, in a parasympathetic state (PCL) corresponding to the symptomatic phase, once subjected to the drugs' action administered by the doctor, it will be stimulated to go to the sympathetic phase where the symptomatology improvement occurs. Ending the cycle of the therapeutic drug, the biological process resumes and the tissue, no longer subjected to the chemical action, returns to parasympathicotonia and, consequently, symptoms will occur again.

If the person is relapsing a 2, 3 or 10 months separation conflict, we can say certainly that therapies will not work; but if he stops relapsing when being subjected to drug therapy, at the end of treatment symptomatology will not represent because the curve will not be activated but will be in normotonia.

13. Cutaneous Allergies

According to the 5 Biological Laws, the so-called "allergies" "manifest":

- in the post-conflict solution (more symptomatic)
- through activation of the conflicting tracks

According to the 1st Biological Law, at the moment of the DHS the individual "records" biologically, but not consciously, all those details present at that time in which he lived the DHS. For example, if I live a DHS producing a biphasic curve, when I'm walking on the bank of a stream, in that moment I will do as a "sensory picture" of everything that surrounds me: the sound of water, odors smells, the temperature, the humidity, the insects, I can hear the voices and much more. From that moment I have set tracks that will be "stored" for a long time or, at least, until they will become aware. Whenever I relive or some tracks related to a precise and already experienced DHS represent, the biphasic curve will be instantly reactivated, thus giving me consequently a symptomatic manifestation that often is appointed as "allergic manifestation".

A real example can help in understanding those events that we call allergies. A young woman reports being allergic to raw tomatoes. She cannot neither touch them with her hands nor eat them; if tomatoes are cooked, nothing happens, but the raw ones trigger an allergic and intense reaction and this situation has been lasting since 18-20 years.

According to the 5 Biological Laws that person lived a DHS where there were tomatoes or by touching them!

In fact, this person was asked to remember a certain intense event experienced prior to her allergy, and she recalled that once upon a child she went into a farmer's garden with her friend to pick tomatoes. The farmer, seeing something moving in the garden, had fired into the air with his rifle and, together with his barking dog, he began running toward the garden. The two girls ran away. Since that time, as reported by the woman, she began to show the "strange allergy." Biologically it has a complete sense. At the moment of the DHS she was holding the tomato and the vegetable produced the track. Whenever she resumed the track, biologically she read it as a danger and the skin reaction was the so called "allergy to tomatoes."

Of course, the common question is: can she now eat tomatoes? The answer is "yes". Asking to the same person what happened in relation to tomatoes, she told me that she went buying them with greater awareness while recalling the fateful event. And she did not show skin reaction any more.

Another example: a child started developing a dermatitis in the areas of the solar plexus and cheeks. Investigating better with his parents, it was revealed that the child had been given a little puppy dog a few weeks before. The child, as soon as possible, laid down on the bed or on the sofa putting the puppy on his stomach and let the animal free of kissing his face (cheeks). Thus far no problem, but then the grandfather started rebuking him not to put the dog on the bed. So the child, having to put the puppy on the ground, suffered a separation conflict. Every time he wrapped his arms around the puppy in the absence of his grandfather, he went into resolution and dermatitis occurred in the area of separation. Since his grandfather was told not to rebuke him again, the "dermatitis" disappeared.

The principle is simple: after a separation conflict the biphasic curve starts. Until the Active Conflict (CA) is present that is the separation is active, the epidermis is more or less dry. When the Conflict Solution (CL) starts, that is a reconciliation takes place with the one who we were separated from, the edematous inflammatory phase occurs which will last in relation to the AC phase duration, in the absence of relapses.

14. The research of conflicts and tracks

Having defined and understood the various phases of the biphasic curve, the behavior of tissue regarding the personal life, we can go to the next step to identify all the important components for the reading of the symptoms in relation to the 5 Biological Laws.

Below, a proposal for useful questions during the research of conflicts and conflicting tracks that have occurred and here below the answer-explanation.

Case of Dermatitis

Questions and answers

What is the symptomatic manifestation?

-    Dermatitis

Which tissue is involved?

-    Epidermis

To what kind of conflict does the involved tissue respond?

-   Conflict of separation

How does that tissue behave according to the 3rd Biological Law?

-   The epidermis derives from the ectoderm and, like all tissues derived from the ectoderm, in CA there is a reduction of tissue and function. The area has a decreased perception, while after the CL tissue and function are restored with increased sensitivity, redness, swollen ... symptomatic phase.

Where does it occur in the body?

-   in the inner part of both the arms. The location of the "injuries" follows the law of laterality or the area where the separation occurred, as in this case.

When did you experience the first event?

-   2 years ago

Where did the first manifestation appear in the body?

-   Also in the same area

Has the symptomatic event changed over time?

- No it has not

How long has this event been lasting?

- since two years

Do symptoms come and go?

- Yes, it looks better, but then gets worse

Have you identified some triggering events or situations?

- Yes and no, but they are not always the same

When does the dermatitis get worse?

- in the weekend, but it does not always occur

When does it seem to get better?

- During the weekdays

These questions are more than enough to look for the triggering event/s.

Through the knowledge of the 5 Biological Laws and the data collected we can assume that this woman, 2 years ago, experienced a conflict of separation from those who she wanted to embrace because the interested areas are the inner part of the arms, most likely from parents (mother and father or brothers-sisters) or from a person close to her, not necessarily of the household. Representing dermatitis with a regular cycle for two years, it means that the person is relapsing, that is to say since 2 years till now she has been meeting (hugs) with these or this person. And it is natural to expect that the dermatitis gets worse when reviewing or reembracing these people. The symptoms, in this case of dermatitis, only occur during the Conflict Solution (CL) that is a positive event, and in dermatitis case it is a reconciliation.

Everything should be checked only by asking question to the involved, such as:

What happened in her life about two years ago?

-   I got married

Where did you live?

-   With my husband at 130 km away from my parents' house

Do you miss your parents?

- Yes a lot, as soon as we can, we go and see them, but working during the week we go on weekends.

Have you noticed, by chance, that the dermatitis gets worse when you go to visit your parents?

- Yes it is! In fact, I have asked several times why this happened. I thought it was the detergent and conditioner used by my mom, but then I saw that I used both of them in my home and I excluded this cause. But I could not understand. Ah ... now everything is clear!

The process, the understanding of the process and simply the practical application may sometimes be difficult, especially in the early stages of the study and application of the 5 Biological Laws. Dr. Hamer did not discover "new things", but he only understood and subsequently codified what we had always lived and had been under our eyes for centuries.

Dr. Hamer understood and verified that the cause of the so-called "disorders" is due to particular events that the individual lives in his existence, in his everyday life, while we have always looked for the causes outwards the human being, towards the viruses, bacteria, fungi, errors, errors of the immune system, age, atmospheric agents ...; thus always, rightly, assuming multifactorial causes as unable of finding the causes of the "disease" in the 98%.

15. The therapy, the treatment

Talking about therapy when we look at reality through the 5 Biological Laws makes no sense. The therapy is already the DHS as said by Dr. Hamer. If I live an acute, dramatic, unexpected event is normal that the autonomic nervous system responds effectively to remedy very quickly. concerning a conflict of separation in sympathicotonia (CA), there is a decrease of tissue and function. This means that the skin of the person who experienced the separation will show a reduction of skin sensitivity, more or less feeble and for the duration of sympathicotonia. This, from the biological point of view, it's great because during the active conflict (CA) of a separation allows me to "feel less" the separation from the person. If I don't feel, I do not suffer. Solving the separation (CL), the involved tissue restores its functionality and, above all, the party involved in PCLA will become hypersensitive even more if we are in a state of refugee. The active refugee always intensifies the symptomatic phase of resolution.

By understanding "why" you are already midway. The clean and clear understanding of the 5 Biological Laws lets us able to understand why, and with greater awareness allows us, very often, if there are the conditions, to get out of relapses or to "move from there". Other times it helps us to predict the "worsening of symptoms" always in relation to an event; or at other times not being able to move, I'll be forced to live the process while listening.

APPENDIX

The Nervous System

The nervous system is anatomically organized as follows:

- **Central Nervous System** (CNS) which comprises the encephalon (brain) and spinal cord (neuraxis): it receives, integrates, and processes the afferent stimuli coming from the Peripheral Nervous System(PNS) which in turn receives the efferent stimuli from the CNS.

- **Peripheral Nervous System** (PNS) consists of cranial nerves and spinal nerves stemming from the spinal cord and it is divided in two main parts:

  - **Somatic Nervous System** (SNS) controlling voluntary responses.

  - **Autonomic Nervous System** (ANS), in charge of involuntary responses, consisting of:

    - **Parasympathetic Nervous System**

    - **Sympathetic Nervous System**

The Autonomic Nervous System, in addition to regulating the homeostasis of the organism, controls all functions of the body that are not normally under conscious control; innervating every tissue, organ and bowel, this system cannot be influenced by will and functions with autonomous mechanisms but still in close mutual collaboration with the Central Nervous System.

The orthosympathetic innervation is traditionally described as a component that performs an escape/attack alert function, mobilizes and organizes energy resources in an emergency or in danger,stimulates the heart and lungs,dilates the bronchi,contracts the arteries and inhibits the digestive system; it prepares the body for physical activity, while the parasympathetic system is a system that allows saving energy, digestion, sleep and rest.

Embriologial Layers

The fertilized cell (zygote) through processes of division, differentiation and growth will generate the foetus.

Embryonic development goes through several stages of segmentation (morula, blastocysts), gastrulation and organogenesis.

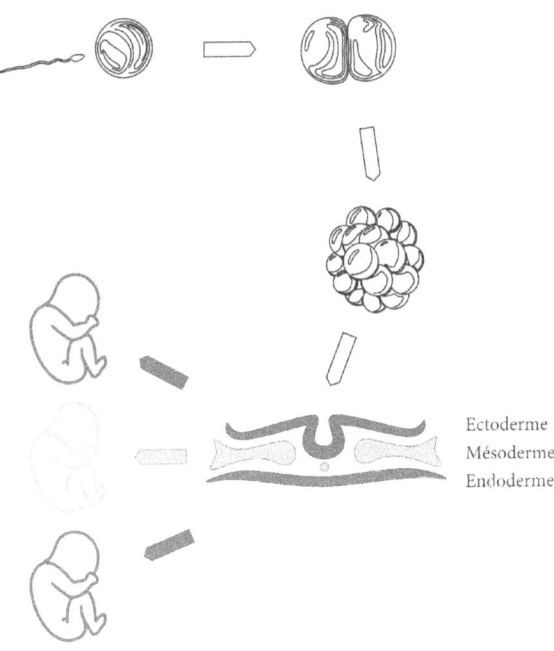

Ectoderme
Mésoderme
Endoderme

In gastrulation, the cells are distributed in three layers of tissue:

- Endoderm

- Mesoderm

- Ectoderm

By subsequent differentiation, all tissues of the body are generated. At the 8th week of gestation, embryonic development is completed to begin organogenesis and the embryo is now called foetus.

CHARTS

The 5 Biological Laws

of **Endodermal origin** tissues

directed by **Cerebral Trunk**

for : **"morsel" conflicts**

Endodermal tissues:

Oral submucosa

Palate

Parotid glands

Sublingual salivary glands

Tonsils

Adenoids *(pharyngeal)*

Lacrimal glands

Iris

Thyroid gland

Posterior pituitary

Middle ear

Eustachian tube

Lower third of the esophagus *(except 2/3 less)*

Alveoli

Greater curvature of the stomach *(except small curvature)*

Liver parenchyma *(except the bile ducts and gallbladder)*

Pancreatic parenchyma *(except pancreatic ducts and Islands of Langerhans)*

Columnar epithelium of the gastro-intestinal

Duodenum *(except the duodenal bulb)*

Small intestine, large intestine and sigma

Inside the navel

Adrenal medulla *(except the adrenal cortex)*

Renal collecting tubules

Rectal submucosa

Trigone of the bladder

Mucosa of the corpus uteri

Bartholin's glands

Fallopian tubes

Ovarian tissue *(except the interstitial tissue)*

Testicular tissue

Prostate

Glands that produce the smegma

Smooth muscle.

The 5 Biological Laws

of **mesodermal** origin tissues

directed by **Cerebellum**

for: **"attack/feeling attacked"** conflicts

Tissues of mesodermal origin:

Derma
Mammary gland (except ducts)
Pericardium
Pleura
Peritoneum
Greater omentum

Tissues of **mesodermal** origin

directed by the **White Matter**

for : **"self-devaluation" conflicts**

Tissues of mesodermal origin:

Connective tissue

Lymphoid tissue *(lymph nodes)*

Tendon tissue

Adipose tissue

Cartilage

Bone

Teeth *(dentin)*

Spleen

Striated muscles

The artery wall

Walls of the veins

Myocardial tissue

Uterine smooth muscle

Muscles of the cervical

Annular sphincter muscles of the neck of the uterus

Muscles *(striated)* of the bladder

Bladder sphincter muscle ring

Smooth muscle of the intestinal tract

Muscles *(striated)* of the rectum

Annular muscles of the anal sphincter

Adrenal cortex

Ovarian interstitial tissue *(excluding parenchyma)*

Testicular interstitial tissue *(excluding parenchyma)*

Renal parenchyma

The 5 Biological Laws

of tissues of **Ectodermal origin**

directed by the **Cerebral Cortex**

for: **"Territorial and separation"** conflicts

Tissues of ectodermal origin:

Epithelium pavimentoso
       Ducts thyroid
       Larynx
       The gill arches
       The milk ducts(breast)
       of the bronchial mucosa
       of the pancreatic ducts
       of biliary ducts
       of the renal pelvis and ureters
       Epidermis
       of the eyelid and conjunctiva
       Tear ducts
       Ducts of the parotid and sublingual glands
Vitreous body, cornea and lens
Tooth enamel
Intima of arteries and coronary veins
Nasal mucosa and paranasal sinuses
Oral mucosa
Mucosa of the upper 2/3of the esophagus

Gastric mucosa(small curvature)

Mucosa of the neck and orifice of the uterus

Vaginal mucosa

Rectal mucosa

Bladder mucosa(excluding the trigone)

Pancreas Cells (alpha and beta)

Periosteum

About the author

Andrea Taddei (Milan 1970, Italy), during the period of his study at the University of Medicine, he learns also different bio-disciplines such as Craniosacral Therapy, Traditional Chinese Medicine, Shiatsu, Ayurvedic Medicine, Yoga and Meditation.[1] Following the abandonment of Academic studies, he devoted full time to the diffusion and study of Craniosacral Therapy. He holds educational seminars and advanced courses on the 5 Biological Laws in Italy and abroad.

The reference site is: www.5biologicallaws.com

Bibliography

English

Dr. Med. Mag. Theol. Ryke Geerd Hamer
Scientific Chart of GNM
Amici di Dirk - Ediciones de la Nueva Medicina S.L.

Andrea Taddei
The 5 Biological Laws and Dr. Hamer's New Medicine
©2012 Andrea Taddei (Sell on Amazon)

Andrea Taddei
The 5 Biological Laws: Bones, Muscles and Articulations.
Dr. Hamer's New Medicine
©2013 Andrea Taddei (Sell on Amazon)

Andrea Taddei
Craniosacral Network Method
©2014 Andrea Taddei (Sell on Amazon)

Spanish

Andrea Taddei
Las 5 Leyes Biológicas y la Nueva Medicina del Doctor Hamer
©2013 Andrea Taddei (Sell on Amazon)

Andrea Taddei

Las 5 Leyes Biologicas: Huesos, Musculos y Articulaciones
La Nueva Medicina del Dr. Hamer
©2013 Andrea Taddei (Sell on Amazon)

Andrea Taddei
Las 5 Leyes Biologicas: La Piel y las Alergias Cutaneas
La Nueva Medicina del Dr. Hamer
©2013 Andrea Taddei (Sell on Amazon)

French

Dr. Med. Mag. Theol. Ryke Geerd Hamer
Tableau scientifique de la Médecine Nouvelle Germanique
Amici di Dirk - Ediciones de la Nueva Medicina S.L.

Andrea Taddei
Les 5 Lois Biologiques et la Médecine Nouvelle du Dr. Hamer
©2012 Andrea Taddei (Sell on Amazon)

Andrea Taddei
Les 5 Lois Biologiques: Os, Muscles et Articulations
La Médecine Nouvelle du Dr. Hamer
©2013 Andrea Taddei (Sell on Amazon)

German

Dr. Med. Mag. Theol. Ryke Geerd Hamer
Wissenschaftliche Tabelle der GNM
Amici di Dirk - Ediciones de la Nueva Medicina S.L.

Dr. Med. Mag. Theol. Ryke Geerd Hamer
Vermächtnis einer Neuen Medizin, Die "Germanische"
Amici di Dirk - Ediciones de la Nueva Medicina S.L.

Dr. Med. Mag. Theol. Ryke Geerd Hamer
Krebs und alle sogenannten "Krankheiten"- kurze Einführung
Amici di Dirk - Ediciones de la Nueva Medicina S.L.

Dr. Med. Mag. Theol. Ryke Geerd Hamer
Aids die Krankheit, die es gar nicht gibt
Amici di Dirk - Ediciones de la Nueva Medicina S.L.

Dr. Med. Mag. Theol. Ryke Geerd Hamer
"Brustkrebs"- Der häufigste Krebs bei Frauen?
Amici di Dirk - Ediciones de la Nueva Medicina S.L.

Dr. Med. Mag. Theol. Ryke Geerd Hamer
Die Archaischen Melodien
Amici di Dirk - Ediciones de la Nueva Medicina S.L.

Italian

Dr. Med. Mag. Theol. Ryke Geerd Hamer
Testamento per una Nuova Medicina Germanica®
©1999 Amici di Dirk, Ediciones de la Nueva Medicina S.L

Dr. Med. Mag. Theol. Ryke Geerd Hamer
Tabella Scientifica della Nuova Medicina Germanica®
©2007 Amici di Dirk, Ediciones de la Nueva Medicina S.L

Dr. Med. Mag. Theol. Ryke Geerd Hamer

Il Capovolgimento Diagnostico
©2003 Amici di Dirk, Ediciones de la Nueva Medicina S.L

Dr. Med. Mag. Theol. Ryke Geerd Hamer
Il Cancro e tutte le cosidette "malattie"
©2003 Amici di Dirk, Ediciones de la Nueva Medicina S.L

Andrea Taddei
Le 5 Leggi Biologiche e la Nuova Medicina del Dr. Hamer
©2012 Andrea Taddei (Sell on Amazon)

Andrea Taddei
Le 5 Leggi Biologiche: Ossa Muscoli e Articolazioni.
La Nuova Medicina del Dr. Hamer
©2013 Andrea Taddei (Sell on Amazon)

Andrea Taddei
Le 5 Leggi Biologiche: La Pelle e le Allergie Cutanee
La Nuova Medicina del Dr. Hamer
©2014 Andrea Taddei (Sell on Amazon)